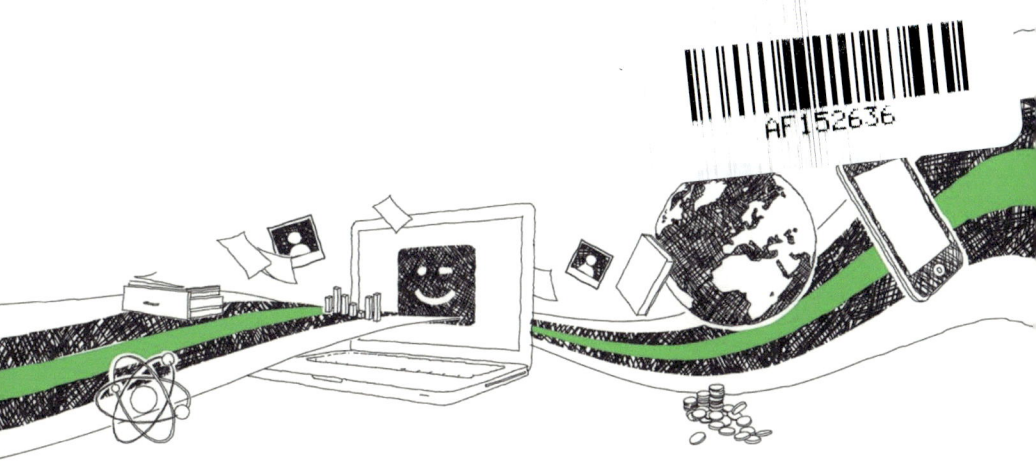

Charles Ross

Genetic modification

GRIN Verlag

Bibliografische Information der Deutschen Nationalbibliothek:

Die Deutsche Bibliothek verzeichnet diese Publikation in der Deutschen National-
bibliografie; detaillierte bibliografische Daten sind im Internet über http://dnb.d-
nb.de/ abrufbar.

Imprint:

Copyright © 2010 GRIN Verlag GmbH
Druck und Bindung: Books on Demand GmbH, Norderstedt Germany
ISBN: 978-3-656-61074-8

This book at GRIN:

http://www.grin.com/en/e-book/269788/genetic-modification

GRIN - Your knowledge has value

Der GRIN Verlag publiziert seit 1998 wissenschaftliche Arbeiten von Studenten, Hochschullehrern und anderen Akademikern als eBook und gedrucktes Buch. Die Verlagswebsite www.grin.com ist die ideale Plattform zur Veröffentlichung von Hausarbeiten, Abschlussarbeiten, wissenschaftlichen Aufsätzen, Dissertationen und Fachbüchern.

Visit us on the internet:

http://www.grin.com/

http://www.facebook.com/grincom

http://www.twitter.com/grin_com

GENETIC MODIFICATION

GENETIC MODIFICATION

Genetic modification is a biotechnology that is used to make new products, in particular new types of crops or organisms < http://www.defra.gov.uk/environment/quality/gm/>. It involves the use of biotechnology techniques to change or alter the genetic make-up of an organism such a plant or animal. All organisms have a make up that is relatively similar, in that each and every organism has its characteristic marked up in the nucleus of its cells in a cellular component known as DNA. In each and every cell, among the billions of cells that make up an organism, contains a cell nucleus that holds this important genetic material known as DNA. The DNA contained in each cell contains mapped out information that controls the functioning of the organism, in addition to carrying the inheritable characteristics that are passed down from one generation of the organism to the next. DNA (deoxyribonucleic acid) is what carries the unique genetic characteristics that conform to each individual. It is these genes that contain instructions to make the building blocks of life in organisms- proteins, starch, oil, fibre or fat that is used within the organism < http://www.csiro.au/Outcomes/Food-and-Agriculture/WhatIsGM.aspx>.

Genetic Modification involves the alteration, elimination or insertion of certain genes in an organism by bio-scientists incorporating genetic engineering techniques to produce an organism with desired characteristics. Genetic modification has been used over the years since its advent to improve on characteristics of organisms such as disease resistant crops, both high and quality yielding crops, the production of industrial and consumer products, the production of hypo-allergic pets, disease resistant animals, transgenic animals (especially mice) used to study human diseases and produce human therapeutics, among others, (Reece, 2004). However, despite the enormous benefits that Genetic Modification has brought to the world today, it has stirred serious ethical debate as to its practice from various viewpoints.

GENETIC MODIFICATION

The science of Genetic Modification has reached great milestones; however, some of its operations have been questioned on ethical grounds. One of the key areas that has been widely attacked and scrutinized on ethical basis is the field of transgenic technology. According to Reece (2004), the process of creating a transgene involves the isolation of a gene of interest from a host organism, which is then altered and subsequent combinations done to it, upon which it is introduced into another organism. Transgenic organisms may either be plant-human combinations, animal-animal, or plant-animal-human combinations. The organism to which a 'new' gene is introduced is what is known as a transgene or chimera, <http://www.actionbioscience.org/biotech/glenn.html>. These transgenic organisms exhibit traits that are completely novel to their species. A good example is the transgenic mice used for development of human therapeutics, (Reece, 2004). These mice are genetically modified to exhibit human characteristics in reaction to diseases. Bioethicists have argued that development of transgenic organisms violates the organisms' intrinsic values, in addition to subjecting these animals to stress.

With the question of transgenic organisms at hand, ethical concerns have been raised as to whether scientists are blurring the lines between natural species, an operation that may alter the natural balance that exists in the natural world as it should be. Bio-scientists have been questioned on whether they are 100% sure of the outcomes of their experiments, while venturing into these unknown realms of science. It has been argued that some of these experiments could result into dangerous uncontrollable species that would be detrimental to human safety, or impact negatively on the environment in the long-run, (Popp, 2012).

Another argument laid forward by ethicists against the development of transgenic organisms is the unknown health risks associated with such productions. By tampering with nature`s natural lines scientists could be breeding softer landing grounds for unknown diseases, or transmission of diseases from one species to another. The health of genetically modified foods is also unknown as no clear testing is done, (Popp, 2012). Humans can not be used to test these foods as they are not taken in controlled amounts, and their long term effects are left unknown.

Another important ethical concern proposed by opponents to genetic modification is the possibility of bio-scientists cloning a human race that could be used as slaves. Several bioethicists have called for a ban on species-altering technology that would be enforced by an international tribunal, < http://www.actionbioscience.org/biotech/glenn.html>. Concerns have been raised over the creation of a slave race of sub-humans whose existence would have unknown implications in the world today. Notwithstanding, the creation of transgenic beings, which have different physique to that of man but with the ability to reason and speak like man, would cause confusion as to what status they should be granted. According to ethicists, this is putting the definition of humans into question. Finally, questions have been raised over the control of such technology. Would the society pre-empt their inborn-nature with that of genetic engineering to produce more intelligent, better-bodied and better looking children? All these ethical concerns have been aired against   the   operation   of   Genetic   Modification <http://www.ornl.gov/sci/techresources/Human_Genome/elsi/gmfood.shtml>.

My take on the ethical concerns towards Genetic Modification leans more to the liberal side. From the great discoveries this field of science has offered, I am personally inclined to support the operation of Genetic Engineering in areas that further human development in medicine and food production to eradicate hunger in the World. However, extensions of these experiments to clone human beings, or similar chimeras should be avoided at all costs as it would be defying human dignity. On the other hand, I strongly advocate for the safe-keeping of

GENETIC MODIFICATION

information regarding Genetic Modification to prevent unauthorized access which may be skewed to serve the mean interests of certain persons, or as a weapon of mass terror.

GENETIC MODIFICATION

Bibliography

< http://www.csiro.au/Outcomes/Food-and-Agriculture/WhatIsGM.aspx>.

< http://www.defra.gov.uk/environment/quality/gm/>.

<http://www.actionbioscience.org/biotech/glenn.html>

<http://www.ornl.gov/sci/techresources/Human_Genome/elsi/gmfood.shtml>

Popp, J. (2012). *The role of biotechnology in a sustainable food supply*. Cambridge: Cambridge
University Press.

Reece, R. J. (2004). *Analysis of Genes and Genomes*. Chichester: John Wiley & Sons.